I0845527

# *"Home Remedies Renaissance: Reviving Ancient Wisdom for Today's Health"*

## *Preface*

Home Remedies Renaissance:

Reviving Ancient Wisdom for Today's Health

In every corner of the world, in kitchens and gardens, the echoes of ancient wisdom linger. Passed down through generations, the remedies that once whispered through the ages are awakening once more. In this age of modern marvels, we find ourselves drawn back to the roots of healing, to the timeless embrace of home remedies.

Welcome to a journey through the age-old tapestry of natural healing. In these pages, we will uncover the treasures of traditional knowledge, breathing life into remedies that have weathered the test of time. As we stand at the crossroads of ancient wisdom and contemporary wellness, we embark on a quest to rekindle the flames of holistic health.

From the soothing balms tucked away in your grandmother's cupboard to the herbs that flourish in your backyard, we invite you to rediscover the healing bounty that surrounds you. Home remedies are not relics of a bygone era but guides to a sustainable and mindful approach to well-being.

As we navigate the labyrinth of health in the 21st century, let this book be your compass. Let the chapters unfold like petals, revealing the richness of nature's apothecary. From the kitchen to the garden, from ancient texts to modern insights, we delve into a resurgence of knowledge that transcends time.

Join us on this odyssey, where age-old wisdom intertwines with the advancements of today. In the Home Remedies Renaissance, we honor the roots that ground us, the remedies that sustain us, and the wisdom that has journeyed through centuries to find its place in the tapestry of our lives.

Embrace the revival, embark on the journey, and let the remedies resonate through your home, your health, and your heart.

May the remedies of yesterday illuminate the path to well-being tomorrow.

With gratitude for the wisdom of generations,

**Akash Gupta**

**Content**

# Roots of Wellness: Exploring Traditional Healing Practices

In this foundational chapter, we delve into the rich tapestry of traditional healing methods that form the roots of wellness. Readers will embark on a journey through time, discovering ancient practices from various cultures that have stood the test of time.

### Unearthing Ancient Wisdom

Explore the origins of traditional healing, from Ayurveda in India to Traditional Chinese Medicine and Indigenous healing practices. Uncover the philosophies that guide these approaches, emphasizing the interconnectedness of mind, body, and spirit.

### Holistic Healing Philosophy

Delve into the holistic approach of traditional healing, understanding how it addresses not just symptoms but the underlying causes of ailments. This section emphasizes the importance of balance and harmony in achieving overall well-being.

### Herbalism Across Cultures

Discover the diverse world of medicinal plants used in different cultures. Highlighting specific herbs with centuries-old reputations for their healing properties, readers will gain insights into the versatile botanical remedies that have been trusted for generations.

### The Wisdom of Healers

Profiles of renowned healers and their contributions to traditional medicine provide a personal touch. From ancient sages to contemporary practitioners, these stories showcase the human connection to healing practices passed down through generations.

### Modern Resurgence of Traditional Healing

Examine the resurgence of interest in traditional healing methods in the modern world. Understand how people are integrating these practices into their lives, seeking alternatives to conventional medicine for a more balanced and personalized approach to health.

### Practical Tips for Embracing Tradition

Offer practical tips for incorporating traditional healing into daily life. From mindfulness practices to simple rituals, readers will learn how to integrate ancient wisdom into their contemporary routines.

By the end of this chapter, readers will have a profound appreciation for the time-honored traditions that underpin holistic health. This sets the stage for the practical and innovative home remedies they'll explore in the chapters to come.

# Garden Pharmacy: Growing and Harvesting Medicinal Herbs

Step into the enchanting world of your own garden transformed into a potent pharmacy. This chapter is a green-thumbed guide to cultivating and harvesting medicinal herbs, empowering readers to create a thriving garden of wellness right at their doorstep.

### Cultivating Healing Spaces

Explore the art of creating a medicinal herb garden, from selecting the right location to designing a layout that maximizes growth. Discover how the very act of cultivating these plants becomes a therapeutic and nurturing experience.

### Herbal Companions

Dive into the symbiotic relationships between different herbs. Learn about companion planting and how certain herbs enhance the growth and potency of their neighboring companions, fostering a harmonious garden ecosystem.

### Essential Medicinal Herbs

Highlight a selection of must-have medicinal herbs, detailing their unique properties and uses. From soothing chamomile and versatile lavender to the powerful echinacea, readers will gain insights into the multifaceted benefits of each herb.

### Seasons of Harvest

Navigate the seasons and understand the optimal times to harvest herbs for maximum potency. This section provides a seasonal calendar, guiding readers on when to pluck the leaves, flowers, or roots of their medicinal plants for various remedies.

### DIY Herbal Remedies

Empower readers with simple yet effective recipes for turning freshly harvested herbs into healing concoctions. From herbal teas and tinctures to infused oils and salves, this section encourages hands-on engagement with the healing potential of the garden.

**Preservation Techniques**

Teach readers how to preserve the bounty of their herbal harvest for year-round use. Explore methods such as drying, freezing, and creating herbal extracts, ensuring a lasting supply of homemade remedies.

**Herbal Wisdom from Around the Globe**

Share stories of how medicinal herbs are revered in different cultures worldwide. Highlight the universal language of plant medicine and the shared appreciation for the healing gifts found in nature.

By the end of this chapter, readers will be inspired to transform their outdoor spaces into vibrant apothecaries, cultivating a personal haven of healing that connects them deeply with the earth's natural remedies.

# Kitchen Alchemy: Transforming Ingredients into Healing Elixirs

Embark on a culinary journey that transcends the ordinary kitchen, turning it into a magical space where everyday ingredients become potent healers. In this chapter, we explore the art of kitchen alchemy, empowering readers to concoct healing elixirs from the heart of their homes.

### The Alchemical Kitchen

Introduce the concept of kitchen alchemy, where simple ingredients undergo transformation into powerful remedies. Discuss the connection between traditional alchemy and the age-old practice of infusing intention into the preparation of healing foods and beverages.

### Healing Spices and Aromatics

Delve into the world of spices and aromatics known for their therapeutic properties. From anti-inflammatory turmeric to digestion-aiding ginger, readers will discover how common kitchen staples can be harnessed for both culinary delight and healing benefits.

**Elixirs for Every Ailment**

Present a curated collection of elixir recipes targeting common ailments. Whether it's a soothing broth for colds, a calming tea for stress, or a digestion-boosting concoction, readers will find a diverse range of elixirs to address various health concerns.

**Mindful Cooking Techniques**

Explore the importance of mindful cooking, emphasizing how the process of preparing food can be as healing as the ingredients themselves. Incorporate techniques such as slow cooking, infusions, and herbal pairings to enhance the therapeutic qualities of meals.

**Intuitive Cooking Practices**

Encourage readers to tap into their intuition while cooking, allowing them to adapt recipes based on personal needs and preferences. This section promotes a holistic approach to nourishment that goes beyond following rigid recipes.

**Culinary Rituals for Well-Being**

Introduce the idea of incorporating mindful rituals into daily cooking practices. From setting positive intentions to expressing gratitude for ingredients, these rituals enhance the healing energy infused into every meal.

**Beyond the Plate: Topical Kitchen Remedies**

Extend the concept of kitchen alchemy beyond ingestion by exploring topical remedies. From honey-based facemasks to coffee scrubs, this section demonstrates how the kitchen can be a source of natural beauty and skincare solutions.

By the end of this chapter, readers will view their kitchen not just as a place for preparing meals but as a sacred space where the alchemy of healing unfolds through the transformative power of everyday ingredients.

# Teas and Tonics: Soothing Beverages for Body and Mind

Indulge in the comforting world of teas and tonics, where the simple act of sipping becomes a ritual of self-care. In this chapter, we explore the therapeutic art of crafting beverages that not only tantalize the taste buds but also nurture body and mind.

### The Art of Tea Blending

Introduce the ancient art of tea blending, guiding readers on creating personalized tea blends tailored to their preferences and health needs. Discuss the diverse world of tea leaves, herbs, and spices that form the foundation of these soothing infusions.

### Healing Infusions for Every Mood

Present a spectrum of tea recipes designed to address various moods and health concerns. From energizing morning blends to calming bedtime teas, readers will discover how to harness the power of herbs to create a diverse repertoire of mood-enhancing infusions.

**Tonic Crafting: Beyond Tea**

Expand the beverage repertoire to include tonics—potent concoctions designed to invigorate and restore balance. Explore the world of herbal tonics, adaptogenic elixirs, and immune-boosting drinks, offering readers a range of options to support their well-being.

**The Ritual of Tea Time**

Highlight the importance of incorporating mindful rituals into tea and tonic consumption. From selecting the perfect teapot to savoring each sip with intention, readers will learn to transform these moments into meditative practices.

**Herb Profiles: Tea's Healing Allies**

Explore the healing properties of specific herbs commonly used in teas and tonics. From chamomile's calming effects to peppermint's digestive benefits, readers will gain a deeper understanding of how each herb contributes to the overall well-being of the body and mind.

**Cold Infusions and Summer Sips**

Adapt tea crafting to different seasons, introducing refreshing cold infusions and summer tonics. Provide recipes that not only quench thirst but also deliver a burst of seasonal vitality.

**Tea for Two: Sharing the Brew**

Encourage the communal aspect of tea and tonic crafting. Whether enjoyed alone for self-reflection or shared with loved ones, emphasize the social and emotional dimensions of these healing beverages.

By the end of this chapter, readers will have not only expanded their beverage-making skills but also cultivated a mindful approach to the act of brewing and sipping, turning everyday moments into opportunities for self-care and rejuvenation.

# Balancing Act: Hormonal Harmony through Natural Remedies

Step into the realm of hormonal health and discover how natural remedies can play a pivotal role in achieving balance. This chapter explores the intricate dance of hormones within the body and offers empowering solutions for fostering harmony through holistic approaches.

### Hormonal Symphony: Understanding the Balance

Provide an accessible yet comprehensive overview of the endocrine system, explaining the role of hormones and their impact on overall well-being. Help readers grasp the delicate balance required for optimal health.

### Nature's Hormone Helpers

Introduce a selection of herbs and plants known for their positive influence on hormonal health. From adaptogenic herbs like ashwagandha to hormone-balancing foods, readers will learn about natural allies that support the body's hormonal equilibrium.

**Nourishing the Endocrine System**

Explore the connection between nutrition and hormonal health. Offer insights into nutrient-rich foods that specifically support the endocrine system, helping readers make informed choices to promote balance from the inside out.

**Mind-Body Practices for Hormonal Harmony**

Highlight the profound impact of stress on hormonal balance and introduce mind-body practices such as yoga, meditation, and deep breathing. Provide practical tips for incorporating these practices into daily routines to mitigate stress and promote hormonal equilibrium.

**Rituals for Hormonal Well-Being**

Encourage the development of mindful rituals that contribute to hormonal health. From morning routines that set a positive tone for the day to bedtime rituals that promote restful sleep, guide readers in creating a nurturing environment for hormonal balance.

**Herbal Formulas for Hormonal Support**

Share specific herbal formulas and remedies designed to address common hormonal imbalances. Whether it's supporting menstrual health, easing menopausal symptoms, or enhancing fertility, readers will find practical solutions rooted in nature.

**Tracking Hormonal Cycles**

Educate readers on the importance of understanding and tracking their hormonal cycles. Provide insights into recognizing signs of imbalance and offer guidance on lifestyle adjustments and remedies to address specific hormonal challenges.

**Hormonal Harmony for Men**

Acknowledge that hormonal balance is crucial for both men and women. Discuss remedies and lifestyle practices that support men's hormonal health, addressing issues such as testosterone balance and prostate health.

By the end of this chapter, readers will have a holistic understanding of hormonal health and a toolkit of natural remedies to promote balance. Empowered with knowledge, they can embark on a journey towards hormonal harmony for enhanced overall well-being.

# Seasonal Serenity: Adapting Remedies for Changing Weather

Embark on a journey through the seasons and discover how to adapt home remedies to embrace the ever-shifting tapestry of weather. This chapter guides readers in crafting a seasonal approach to wellness, ensuring that remedies align with the unique challenges and opportunities each season presents.

### Seasonal Wisdom in Traditional Medicine

Explore how traditional healing practices have long recognized the influence of seasons on health. Introduce the concept of adapting remedies based on the principles of Ayurveda, Traditional Chinese Medicine, and other ancient systems.

### Spring Renewal: Cleansing and Vitality

Guide readers through remedies suited for spring, focusing on cleansing and revitalizing the body. From detoxifying teas to invigorating herbal infusions, help

readers transition from winter lethargy to the energy of
spring.

**Summer Coolers: Hydration and Sun Support**

Highlight remedies that keep the body cool and hydrated
during the heat of summer. Explore refreshing drinks,
sunburn soothers, and tips for maintaining balance in the
face of summer's challenges.

**Autumn Harvest: Immune Boosters and Comfort**

Navigate the transition to fall with remedies that support
the immune system and provide comfort. Showcase
seasonal herbs and foods that offer a fortifying embrace
against the onset of colder weather.

**Winter Wellness: Nourishment and Resilience**

Explore remedies that nurture the body during the winter
months. From immune-boosting broths to soothing
herbal teas, provide readers with tools to fortify
themselves against winter's cold and flu season.

**Seasonal Rituals for Well-Being**

Encourage the adoption of seasonal rituals that promote
overall well-being. Whether it's a spring cleanse, summer

outdoor activities, autumn reflection, or winter self-care practices, emphasize the importance of aligning with the rhythms of nature.

**Garden-to-Table Remedies**

Inspire readers to leverage their gardens for seasonal remedies. Discuss planting strategies that align with the changing needs of each season, creating a dynamic garden pharmacy that evolves with nature.

**Balancing Indoor Environments**

Address the challenges of spending more time indoors during certain seasons. Provide remedies for maintaining indoor air quality, combating seasonal affective disorder (SAD), and creating a cozy, nurturing space.

By the end of this chapter, readers will not only have a seasonal toolkit of remedies but also a deeper appreciation for the cyclical nature of wellness. Armed with this knowledge, they can proactively adapt their self-care practices to thrive in harmony with the changing seasons.

# Home Spa Essentials: DIY Beauty Treatments for Radiant Skin

Indulge in the luxury of a spa experience right within the comfort of your home. This chapter unveils the secrets of DIY beauty treatments using natural ingredients, allowing readers to pamper themselves and cultivate radiant skin with simple yet effective home spa rituals.

### The Art of Home Spa

Introduce the concept of creating a spa-like atmosphere at home, emphasizing the therapeutic benefits of self-care rituals. Discuss the importance of nurturing the skin as part of overall well-being.

### Kitchen Elixirs for Glowing Skin

Explore common kitchen ingredients that double as potent beauty elixirs. From honey and yogurt masks to avocado and coconut oil treatments, guide readers in harnessing the power of nature to nourish and revitalize their skin.

**Herbal Infusions for External Radiance**

Introduce the use of herbal infusions in skincare. From chamomile toners to rose petal baths, showcase how botanicals can be incorporated into beauty routines for their soothing and rejuvenating properties.

**DIY Facial Massage Techniques**

Teach readers simple facial massage techniques that promote circulation, reduce tension, and enhance the absorption of skincare products. Provide step-by-step instructions for a relaxing facial massage routine.

**Natural Exfoliation: Scrubs and Masks**

Explore the world of natural exfoliants and masks to rejuvenate the skin. From sugar scrubs to clay masks, offer recipes that cater to different skin types and concerns, promoting a radiant complexion.

**Essential Oils for Skincare**

Highlight the use of essential oils in skincare routines. Discuss the benefits of popular essential oils such as lavender, tea tree, and rosemary, guiding readers on safe and effective ways to incorporate them into their beauty rituals.

**Hydration Hacks: DIY Moisturizers**

Guide readers in creating their own moisturizers using nourishing ingredients. From shea butter balms to aloe vera gel blends, empower them to customize skincare products that address their unique skin needs.

**Mindful Beauty Practices**

Encourage the integration of mindfulness into beauty routines. Discuss the concept of mindful skincare, emphasizing the connection between self-care rituals and mental well-being.

**Eco-Friendly Beauty: DIY Packaging**

Extend the concept of home spa to include eco-friendly practices. Share ideas for sustainable and reusable packaging for DIY beauty products, promoting an eco-conscious approach to self-care.

By the end of this chapter, readers will have transformed their skincare routine into a holistic and rejuvenating practice. Armed with the knowledge of DIY beauty treatments, they can revel in the luxurious experience of a home spa while nurturing radiant and healthy skin.

# Mindful Eating, Mindful Healing: Food as Medicine

Embark on a transformative journey where each bite becomes an opportunity for nourishment and healing. This chapter explores the concept of mindful eating, emphasizing the profound impact of food choices on overall well-being and offering practical insights into harnessing food as medicine.

### The Mind-Body Connection

Delve into the intricate relationship between the mind and the digestive system. Explore how mindful eating practices can positively influence digestion, nutrient absorption, and overall health.

### The Power of Intuitive Eating

Introduce the concept of intuitive eating, emphasizing the importance of listening to the body's cues and cultivating a deeper awareness of hunger and fullness. Guide readers in reconnecting with their innate ability to make nourishing food choices.

**Whole Foods for Whole Health**

Highlight the benefits of consuming whole, unprocessed foods. Showcase the healing potential of nutrient-dense fruits, vegetables, whole grains, and plant-based proteins, encouraging readers to build a foundation of well-being through their daily food choices.

**Healing Foods and Superfoods**

Explore specific foods celebrated for their healing properties. From antioxidant-rich berries to inflammation-reducing turmeric, provide a comprehensive guide to incorporating these nutritional powerhouses into everyday meals.

**Culinary Medicine: Cooking for Health**

Encourage readers to view cooking as a form of medicine. Discuss cooking techniques that preserve the nutritional value of ingredients and offer tips for creating balanced, flavorful meals that promote healing from within.

**Ayurvedic Nutrition Principles**

Introduce Ayurvedic principles of nutrition, emphasizing the importance of balancing the body's unique constitution through dietary choices. Guide readers in identifying their dosha and adapting their diet accordingly for optimal well-being.

### Mindful Meal Planning

Provide practical tips for mindful meal planning, including grocery shopping strategies, batch cooking ideas, and creating a harmonious eating environment. Empower readers to approach mealtime with intention and mindfulness.

### Seasonal Eating for Vibrancy

Explore the concept of seasonal eating and its impact on health. Discuss the nutritional benefits of aligning dietary choices with the seasons, providing guidance on incorporating a variety of fresh, seasonal produce into meals.

### Food Rituals for Emotional Well-Being

Acknowledge the emotional dimension of eating and introduce rituals that promote emotional well-being. From gratitude practices to mindful eating exercises, guide readers in cultivating a positive relationship with food.

By the end of this chapter, readers will have gained a profound understanding of the healing potential of mindful eating. Empowered with practical tools and insights, they can embark on a journey where each meal becomes a mindful act of self-care and a source of holistic nourishment.

# Sleep Sanctuary: Herbal Solutions for Restful Nights

Immerse yourself in the world of restful sleep and create a sanctuary that promotes deep, rejuvenating rest. This chapter explores the significance of sleep for overall well-being and offers herbal solutions to enhance the quality of sleep, ensuring readers wake up refreshed and revitalized.

### The Importance of Quality Sleep

Begin by highlighting the critical role sleep plays in physical and mental health. Discuss the various aspects of well-being that are positively impacted by consistent, high-quality sleep.

### Creating a Sleep-Inducing Environment

Guide readers in transforming their sleep space into a serene sanctuary. Discuss elements such as comfortable bedding, calming colors, and the elimination of electronic distractions to foster an environment conducive to restful sleep.

### Herbs for Relaxation and Stress Reduction

Explore herbs renowned for their relaxation-inducing properties. From chamomile and valerian to passionflower, provide insights into how these herbs can be incorporated into teas, tinctures, or aromatherapy to promote relaxation and ease stress.

### Bedtime Rituals for Tranquility

Introduce bedtime rituals that signal the body and mind that it's time to unwind. From gentle stretches to calming breathing exercises, empower readers to establish a routine that promotes relaxation and prepares them for a restful night's sleep.

### Herbal Teas for Sleep Support

Share a curated selection of herbal tea recipes specifically designed to promote sleep. Discuss the benefits of ingredients such as lavender, lemon balm, and skullcap, guiding readers in crafting soothing blends to enjoy before bedtime.

### Aromatherapy for Sleep

Explore the use of essential oils in creating a restful sleep atmosphere. Provide recommendations for calming scents such as lavender and chamomile, and guide readers on incorporating aromatherapy into their pre-sleep rituals.

### Mindful Digital Detox before Bed

Address the impact of screen time on sleep quality. Offer tips for implementing a mindful digital detox before bedtime, emphasizing the importance of disconnecting from electronic devices to promote relaxation.

### Sleep Hygiene Practices

Educate readers on the principles of good sleep hygiene. Discuss factors such as maintaining a consistent sleep schedule, creating a comfortable sleep environment, and avoiding stimulants close to bedtime.

### Herbal Solutions for Sleep Disorders

Address common sleep disorders such as insomnia and restless legs syndrome. Provide herbal remedies and lifestyle tips tailored to specific sleep challenges, empowering readers to find personalized solutions.

By the end of this chapter, readers will have gained a comprehensive understanding of the holistic approach to achieving restful sleep. Armed with herbal solutions and mindful practices, they can create a sleep sanctuary that supports their journey to a night of deep, rejuvenating rest.

# "Spiritual Healing at Home: Finding Inner Peace through Rituals"

Embark on a soul-nourishing journey as we explore the intersection of spirituality and home-based rituals. This chapter delves into the practices that foster inner peace, mindfulness, and a sense of connection with the divine, allowing readers to create a sacred space within their homes.

### The Sacred Space Within

Introduce the concept of a personal sacred space within the home. Discuss the importance of creating a physical and energetic environment that promotes tranquility and serves as a haven for spiritual practices.

### Rituals for Mindful Beginnings and Endings

Guide readers in crafting rituals to mark the beginning and end of each day. Whether it's a morning meditation or an evening gratitude practice, encourage the incorporation of mindful rituals into daily routines.

### Altars and Sacred Symbols

Explore the use of altars and sacred symbols as focal points for spiritual practices. Discuss how carefully chosen objects, images, and symbols can serve as reminders of higher purpose and create a tangible connection to the divine.

### Meditation Practices for Inner Stillness

Introduce various meditation techniques to cultivate inner stillness. From mindfulness meditation to loving-kindness meditation, provide guidance on finding a practice that resonates with each reader's spiritual journey.

### Connecting with Nature Spirituality

Explore the spiritual significance of nature and guide readers in creating a connection with the natural world. Discuss practices such as nature walks, garden meditations, and rituals that honor the cycles of the Earth.

### Sacred Sounds and Mantras

Discuss the transformative power of sound in spiritual practices. Introduce mantras, chants, or sound bowls that can be incorporated into rituals to elevate vibrations and deepen the spiritual experience.

### Rituals for Healing and Renewal

Guide readers in creating rituals specifically focused on healing and renewal. Whether it's energy-clearing practices, healing visualizations, or ceremonies for letting go, empower readers to embark on a journey of spiritual renewal.

### Soulful Journaling and Reflection

Encourage reflective practices such as journaling to deepen spiritual awareness. Provide prompts and exercises that guide readers in exploring their inner landscapes, fostering self-discovery and spiritual growth.

### Rituals for Connection and Community

Explore the spiritual dimension of human connection. Discuss practices that foster a sense of community, whether it's through shared rituals with loved ones, group meditations, or virtual gatherings with like-minded individuals.

**Living with Intention**

Wrap up the chapter by emphasizing the importance of living with intention. Discuss how aligning daily actions with spiritual values contributes to a sense of purpose, fulfillment, and an enduring connection with the sacred.

By the end of this chapter, readers will have a toolkit of spiritual practices that can be seamlessly integrated into their home life, fostering a sense of inner peace, mindfulness, and a profound connection with the spiritual dimensions of existence.

# "Roots to Rise: Yoga and Movement for Holistic Well-Being"

Embark on a transformative journey of self-discovery and holistic well-being through the ancient practice of yoga and mindful movement. This chapter explores the multifaceted benefits of yoga, guiding readers to cultivate physical strength, mental clarity, and spiritual connection within the comfort of their homes.

### The Essence of Yoga Philosophy

Introduce the foundational principles of yoga philosophy, emphasizing the union of mind, body, and spirit. Discuss concepts such as mindfulness, breath awareness, and the pursuit of self-realization as guiding principles for the practice.

### Yoga Asana: Building Physical Strength

Guide readers through a series of yoga asanas (poses) that cater to different fitness levels. From grounding poses like Mountain Pose to strength-building postures like Warrior sequences, empower readers to establish a personalized yoga practice.

### Mindful Movement Beyond Asana

Expand the scope of mindful movement beyond traditional yoga poses. Introduce practices such as tai chi, qigong, or simple stretching routines that enhance flexibility, balance, and overall physical well-being.

### Breathwork for Mind-Body Connection

Explore the transformative power of breathwork in cultivating mindfulness and reducing stress. Introduce pranayama techniques such as deep belly breathing, alternate nostril breathing, and breath awareness to foster a profound mind-body connection.

### Yoga Nidra for Deep Relaxation

Introduce the practice of Yoga Nidra, a guided meditation for deep relaxation. Discuss the benefits of this practice in reducing stress, enhancing sleep, and promoting overall mental well-being.

**Creating a Home Yoga Sanctuary**

Guide readers in establishing a dedicated space for their home yoga practice. Discuss the importance of creating an environment that inspires focus, tranquility, and a sense of sacredness.

**Mindful Movement for Emotional Balance**

Explore the role of mindful movement in emotional regulation. Discuss how yoga and other movement practices can serve as outlets for self-expression and contribute to emotional balance and resilience.

**Yoga for Every Body: Inclusivity and Adaptability**

Emphasize the inclusivity of yoga by discussing variations and modifications suitable for diverse body types and abilities. Encourage readers to embrace a yoga practice that suits their individual needs and capabilities.

**Integrating Yoga Philosophy into Daily Life**

Discuss ways to integrate yoga philosophy into daily life beyond the mat. Explore concepts such as mindfulness in daily activities, conscious eating, and the cultivation of compassion as extensions of the yoga practice.

**Building a Sustainable Yoga Practice**

Offer guidance on building a sustainable and evolving yoga practice. Discuss the importance of consistency, gradual progression, and self-compassion in maintaining a lifelong relationship with yoga and mindful movement.

By the end of this chapter, readers will have gained a comprehensive understanding of the transformative potential of yoga and mindful movement. Empowered with practical insights, they can embark on a journey of self-exploration and holistic well-being, fostering a harmonious balance of mind, body, and spirit.

# "Green Cleaning: Eco-Friendly Solutions for a Healthy Home"

Step into a toxin-free realm by embracing green cleaning practices that not only foster a healthy home environment but also contribute to a sustainable future. This chapter explores eco-friendly cleaning solutions, empowering readers to detoxify their living spaces using simple, natural ingredients.

### Understanding the Impact of Conventional Cleaners

Discuss the potential health hazards associated with common household cleaning products. Explore the impact of harsh chemicals on indoor air quality, respiratory health, and the environment, motivating readers to seek safer alternatives.

### Essential Ingredients for Green Cleaning

Introduce a range of natural ingredients that serve as the backbone of green cleaning solutions. From baking soda and vinegar to essential oils, empower readers to assemble a basic toolkit for effective and environmentally friendly cleaning.

### Multipurpose DIY Cleaners

Provide recipes for versatile DIY cleaners that can be used across various surfaces in the home. From all-purpose surface sprays to floor and glass cleaners, guide readers in creating effective, non-toxic alternatives to commercial products.

### The Art of Natural Deodorizing

Explore natural methods for deodorizing living spaces. Introduce techniques such as using citrus peels, baking soda, and essential oils to neutralize odors, leaving homes smelling fresh without the need for artificial fragrances.

### Eco-Friendly Cleaning Tools and Accessories

Discuss sustainable and reusable cleaning tools that complement green cleaning practices. From microfiber cloths to bamboo scrub brushes, guide readers in making eco-conscious choices for their cleaning routines.

**Green Laundry Practices**

Extend green cleaning to the laundry room. Discuss eco-friendly laundry detergents, natural fabric softeners, and tips for air-drying clothes to reduce energy consumption and environmental impact

# "From Stress to Serenity: Stress Management with Natural Remedies"

Embark on a journey of self-discovery and resilience as we explore natural remedies for managing stress and cultivating serenity. This chapter delves into holistic approaches that empower readers to navigate life's challenges with grace, harnessing the healing power of nature and mindful practices.

### The Impact of Stress on Health

Discuss the physiological and psychological effects of stress on the body and mind. Explore the interconnectedness of stress with various health issues, motivating readers to prioritize stress management for overall well-being.

### Holistic Approaches to Stress Reduction

Introduce the concept of holistic stress reduction, emphasizing the interconnectedness of mental, emotional, and physical well-being. Discuss the role of lifestyle changes, mindfulness practices, and natural remedies in creating a comprehensive approach to stress management.

### Herbal Allies for Stress Relief

Explore herbs renowned for their stress-relieving properties. From adaptogens like ashwagandha to calming herbs such as chamomile and passionflower, provide insights into the natural remedies that can soothe the nervous system and promote relaxation.

### Mindfulness Meditation for Stress Resilience

Guide readers in establishing a mindfulness meditation practice for stress resilience. Discuss techniques such as mindful breathing, body scan meditation, and loving-kindness meditation, offering practical tips for integrating mindfulness into daily life.

### Aromatherapy for Relaxation

Explore the use of essential oils in aromatherapy for stress relief. Discuss calming scents such as lavender, bergamot, and frankincense, and guide readers on incorporating aromatherapy into their routines to create moments of tranquility.

### Stress-Busting Nutrition

Discuss the impact of nutrition on stress levels. Explore stress-busting foods and nutrients, such as omega-3 fatty acids, magnesium, and vitamin B, providing practical dietary tips to support the body during times of stress.

### Creating a Serene Home Environment

Guide readers in transforming their living spaces into sanctuaries of serenity. Discuss the importance of decluttering, creating calming corners, and incorporating natural elements to foster a sense of peace within the home.

### Movement Practices for Stress Release

Introduce movement practices that release tension and promote relaxation. From gentle yoga sequences to tai chi movements, empower readers to incorporate mindful movement into their routines for stress relief.

### Journaling for Emotional Release

Encourage the therapeutic practice of journaling for emotional release. Provide prompts and exercises that guide readers in expressing and processing their emotions, contributing to a greater sense of self-awareness and resilience.

### Rituals for Stressful Moments

Guide readers in creating rituals for moments of stress. Whether it's a calming tea ritual, a brief meditation break, or a nature walk, empower readers to establish go-to practices that offer solace during challenging times.

### Seeking Professional Support

Discuss the importance of seeking professional support when needed. Provide information on therapy, counseling, and other resources that can offer guidance and assistance during times of heightened stress.

By the end of this chapter, readers will have a toolkit of natural remedies and holistic practices to navigate stress and cultivate serenity in their lives. Empowered with these tools, they can face life's challenges with resilience, fostering a sense of balance and well-being.

# "Immune-Boosting Bounty: Fortifying Your Defenses Naturally"

Unlock the secrets of fortifying your body's defenses through a bounty of natural immune-boosting practices. This chapter is a holistic guide to harnessing the power of nature to enhance your immune system and promote overall well-being.

### Understanding the Immune System

Overview of the Immune System:  Provide a foundational understanding of the immune system, explaining its vital role in protecting the body from infections and illnesses.

The Immune System's Complexity: Explore the intricate network of cells, tissues, and organs that collaborate to defend the body against pathogens.

### Nutrient-Rich Foods for Immunity

Essential Vitamins and Minerals: Delve into the essential nutrients that play a key role in supporting immune function, including vitamin C, vitamin D, zinc, and antioxidants.

Immune-Boosting Foods

Present a diverse array of foods rich in immune-supporting nutrients, such as citrus fruits, leafy greens, berries, nuts, and seeds.

## Herbal Allies in Immune Health

Exploration of Immune-Boosting Herbs: Introduce a variety of herbs celebrated for their immune-enhancing properties, such as echinacea, elderberry, astragalus, and medicinal mushrooms.

Incorporating Herbs into Daily Life: Provide practical tips on incorporating immune-boosting herbs into teas, tinctures, and daily meals.

### Functional Foods and Superfoods

Superfoods for Immune Resilience: Highlight the role of superfoods like turmeric, ginger, garlic, and green tea in providing additional immune support.

Functional Foods: Explore the concept of functional foods that offer both nutritional value and potential health benefits for the immune system.

**Creating Immune-Boosting Meals**

Balanced and Nourishing Recipes: Provide a collection of immune-boosting recipes that integrate a variety of nutrient-dense ingredients.

Meal Planning for Immunity: Guide readers in structuring their meals to include a variety of immune-supportive foods throughout the week.

**Lifestyle Practices for Immune Well-being**

Quality Sleep for Immune Support: Emphasize the importance of sufficient and restful sleep in supporting immune function.

Stress Management Techniques:   Introduce stress-reducing practices, such as meditation, yoga, and deep breathing exercises, to promote overall immune resilience.

**Physical Activity and Immune Function**

Benefits of Regular Exercise: Explore how physical activity contributes to overall health and supports immune function.

Choosing Immune-Friendly Exercises: Provide guidance on selecting exercises that enhance immune health without causing excessive stress on the body.

**Holistic Hygiene and Immune Health**

Proper Hygiene Practices: Emphasize the significance of good hygiene, including regular handwashing and maintaining a clean living environment, in preventing infections.

Balancing Cleanliness: Discuss the idea of maintaining a balanced, not overly sterile, environment to allow the immune system to develop resilience.


**Mind-Body Connection and Immunity**

Interconnectedness of Mental and Physical Well-being: Explore the link between mental and immune health, emphasizing practices like mindfulness and relaxation techniques.

Holistic Approaches: Introduce holistic approaches that consider the mind-body connection for comprehensive immune support.


**Environmental Considerations**

Reducing Environmental Exposures: Discuss strategies for minimizing exposure to environmental factors that can compromise immune health, such as pollutants and toxins.

**Creating a Healthy Living Space:** Provide tips for creating a home environment that supports immune resilience.

**Empowering Readers for Immune Wellness**

Integrating Immune Practices into Daily Life: Offer practical tips for seamlessly integrating immune-boosting practices into everyday routines.

Empowerment Through Knowledge: Empower readers with the knowledge and tools to take charge of their immune health and well-being.

By the end of this chapter, readers will have gained a thorough understanding of natural immune-boosting practices and a practical roadmap for incorporating these strategies into their daily lives. Empowered with a bounty of nature's offerings, they can fortify their defenses and nurture overall well-being.

# "Spiritual Healing at Home: Finding Inner Peace through Rituals"

Embark on a transformative journey of spiritual exploration within the comfort of your home. This chapter is a guide to cultivating inner peace, mindfulness, and a profound connection with the divine through a series of meaningful rituals.

### The Sacred Space Within

Creating a Personal Sanctuary:* Explore the concept of a sacred space within the home, emphasizing the importance of a dedicated area for spiritual practices.

Fostering Tranquility: Discuss how the physical and energetic environment of the sacred space contributes to a sense of peace and mindfulness.

### Rituals for Mindful Beginnings and Endings

Morning and Evening Practices: Guide readers in crafting rituals to mark the beginning and end of each day, fostering mindfulness and setting positive intentions.

Gratitude Practices: Introduce gratitude rituals as a way to cultivate a positive and appreciative mindset.

### Altars and Sacred Symbols

Symbolic Representation: Explore the use of altars and sacred symbols as focal points for spiritual practices.

Choosing Meaningful Objects: Discuss the significance of carefully chosen objects, images, and symbols in creating a tangible connection to the divine.

### Meditation Practices for Inner Stillness:

Mindfulness Meditation: Introduce various meditation techniques, such as mindfulness and breath awareness, to cultivate inner stillness.

Guided Meditations: Provide resources for guided meditations that cater to different spiritual journeys.

### Connecting with Nature Spirituality:

Nature as a Spiritual Guide: Explore the spiritual significance of nature and guide readers in creating a connection with the natural world.

Outdoor Practices: Discuss nature walks, garden meditations, and rituals that honor the cycles of the Earth.

**Sacred Sounds and Mantras:**

Transformative Power of Sound: Discuss the use of sound, such as mantras, chants, or sound bowls, in elevating vibrations and enhancing spiritual experiences.

Incorporating Sound into Rituals: Provide practical tips for integrating sacred sounds into daily spiritual rituals.

**Rituals for Healing and Renewal:**

Energy-Clearing Practices: Guide readers in creating rituals focused on energy clearing and healing.

Ceremonies for Letting Go: Explore rituals that facilitate the process of letting go and renewal.

**Soulful Journaling and Reflection:**

Journaling Practices: Encourage reflective practices, such as journaling, to deepen spiritual awareness.

Prompts for Self-Discovery: Provide prompts and exercises that guide readers in exploring their inner landscapes.

**Rituals for Connection and Community:**

Shared Spiritual Practices: Explore the spiritual dimension of human connection.

Virtual Gatherings: Discuss the potential for virtual gatherings and shared rituals with like-minded individuals.

**Living with Intention:**

Aligning Actions with Values: Emphasize the importance of living with intention by aligning daily actions with spiritual values.

Fostering a Sense of Purpose: Discuss how intentional living contributes to a sense of purpose and fulfillment.

By the end of this chapter, readers will have a toolkit of spiritual practices that can be seamlessly integrated into their home life. Whether new to spiritual exploration or seasoned practitioners, they will find guidance in fostering inner peace, mindfulness, and a profound connection with the spiritual dimensions of existence.

www.ingramcontent.com/pod-product-compliance
Lightning Source LLC
Chambersburg PA
CBHW031333250726
48656CB00005B/2109